Table of Contents

BARIATRIC DIET

After weight-loss surgery, it will take time for your body to heal. As your body recovers from surgery, it's essential for you to follow the specific eating guidelines given to you by your bariatric surgeon or dietitian. The bariatric diet for recovery is set to ensure that your body heals properly and obtains adequate nutrition.

BARIATRIC DIET RECIPES

1. Crispy Oven-Roasted Rosemary Chicken with Sausage and Potatoes

Prep Time: 20 mins

Total Time: 1 hr 20 mins

Servings: 6

Ingredients

- ¼ cup olive oil
- 1 pound bratwurst links, cut into 1/2 inch slices
- 2 ½ pounds chicken pieces
- 1 pinch kosher salt to taste
- 2 pounds potatoes, cut into 1-inch chunks
- 2 tablespoons extra-virgin olive oil
- 2 ½ tablespoons fresh rosemary leaves, chopped
- 1 teaspoon red wine vinegar

Directions

1. Preheat oven to 450 degrees F (230 degrees C). Prepare a large baking dish with cooking spray.

2. Pour half of the olive oil into a large skillet over medium heat. Cook the bratwurst in the hot oil until browned on both sides, about 5 minutes; set aside. Add the remaining olive oil to the skillet and return to heat; brown the chicken pieces in the hot oil 7 to 10 minutes; season with salt while cooking; set aside and return the skillet to heat. Heat the potatoes in the skillet until lightly browned. Arrange potatoes, chicken, and bratwurst in the prepared baking dish; season with salt and drizzle with 2 tablespoons olive oil; sprinkle with about half of the chopped rosemary.

3. Roast in the preheated oven 15 minutes. Turn each piece of chicken over and stir the potatoes and sausage. Sprinkle the remaining rosemary and the red wine vinegar over the dish; cook another 15 minutes.

2. Best Salmon Bake

2. Best Salmon Bake

Prep Time: 15 mins

Total Time: 35 mins

Servings: 2

Ingredients

- 1 (1 pound) salmon fillet, halved
- 1 small tomato, chopped
- 5 green onions, chopped
- ¼ teaspoon salt
- ¼ teaspoon pepper

Directions

1. Preheat the oven to 350 degrees F (175 degrees C).
2. Place salmon on a lightly oiled sheet pan or in a shallow baking dish, folding under thin outer edges of fillets for even cooking. Top salmon with chopped tomatoes and green onions, and season with salt and pepper.

3. Cook salmon in the preheated oven, uncovered, until fish flakes easily with a fork, about 20 minutes.

Prep Time: 10 mins

Total Time: 1 hr

Servings: 4

Ingredients

- 4 pounds skin-on, bone-in chicken thighs
- 3 russet potatoes, peeled and quartered
- ½ cup fresh lemon juice
- ½ cup olive oil
- 6 cloves garlic, minced
- 1 tablespoon dried oregano
- 1 tablespoon kosher salt
- 1 teaspoon dried rosemary
- 1 teaspoon freshly ground black pepper
- 1 pinch cayenne pepper
- 1 cup chicken broth, divided
- 1 teaspoon chopped fresh oregano, or to taste

Directions

1. Preheat the oven to 425 degrees F (220 degrees C). Lightly oil a large roasting pan.
2. Place chicken and potatoes in a large bowl. Add lemon juice, olive oil, garlic, dried oregano, salt, rosemary, black pepper, and cayenne. Toss until chicken and potatoes are evenly coated.
3. Place chicken pieces skin-side up in the prepared pan. Tuck potato pieces around chicken. Drizzle with 2/3 cup chicken broth. Spoon any remaining marinade from the bowl over chicken and potatoes.
4. Bake in the preheated oven for 20 minutes. Toss chicken and potatoes, then place chicken skin-side up again.
5. Continue baking until chicken is browned and cooked through, about 25 minutes more; an instant-read thermometer inserted near the bone should register 165 degrees F (74 degrees C).
6. Transfer chicken to a serving platter and keep warm; leave potatoes in the pan.

7. Turn on the broiler, or set oven to highest heat. Toss potatoes again to coat in pan juices. Place the pan under the broiler and broil until potatoes are crisped, about 3 minutes.

8. Transfer potatoes to the platter with chicken.

9. Place the roasting pan on the stovetop over medium heat. Add the remaining 1/3 cup chicken broth and scrape up browned bits from the bottom of the pan. Strain pan juices over chicken and potatoes. Sprinkle with fresh oregano.

4. Vegan Green Bean, Tomato, and Basil Sheet Pan Dinner

Prep Time: 10 mins

Total Time: 55 mins

Servings: 4

Ingredients

- 2 cups baby potatoes
- 3 tablespoons olive oil, divided
- 2 cups cherry tomatoes
- 2 cups 1-inch cut fresh green beans
- 4 cloves garlic, minced
- 2 teaspoons dried basil
- 1 teaspoon flaked sea salt
- 1 (15 ounce) can garbanzo beans, drained and rinsed
- 2 teaspoons olive oil, or to taste
- salt and ground black pepper to taste

Directions

1. Preheat the oven to 425 degrees F (220 degrees C). Line a jelly roll pan with aluminum foil.
2. Toss potatoes with 1 tablespoon olive oil in a medium bowl. Pour into the prepared pan.
3. Roast in the preheated oven until tender, about 30 minutes.
4. Toss cherry tomatoes, green beans, garlic, basil, and sea salt with 2 tablespoons olive oil.
5. Remove potatoes from the oven, push them to one side of the pan, and add the tomato and green bean mixture. Roast until tomatoes start to wilt, 15 to 20 minutes more.
6. Remove from the oven and pour into a serving dish. Stir in garbanzo beans, add 2 teaspoons olive oil, and season with salt and pepper.

5. Sheet Pan Shrimp Fajitas

Prep Time: 20 mins

Total Time: 30 mins

Servings: 8

Ingredients

- 1 (1 ounce) package fajita seasoning
- 1 tablespoon olive oil
- 1 ½ pounds raw shrimp, peeled and deveined
- 1 red bell pepper, sliced into strips
- 1 yellow bell pepper, sliced into strips
- 1 red onion, sliced into strips
- 1 jalapeno pepper, sliced into rings

Directions

1. Preheat the oven to 450 degrees F (230 degrees C).
2. Mix fajita seasoning and olive oil together in a large bowl. Add shrimp; toss to coat.

3. Lay out seasoned shrimp in a single layer on a baking sheet. Add bell peppers, red onion, and jalapeño; mix with shrimp and spread out evenly.

4. Roast in the preheated oven until shrimp are opaque, 8 to 10 minutes. Transfer shrimp to a serving plate.

5. Broil pepper mixture until lightly blackened, 2 to 3 minutes. Transfer to the serving plate with shrimp.

4. Sausage, Peppers, Onions, and Potato Bake

Prep Time: 20 mins

Total Time: 1 hr

Servings: 8

Ingredients

- 2 teaspoons olive oil
- 2 pounds Italian sausage links, cut into 2-inch pieces
- ¼ cup olive oil
- 4 large potatoes, peeled and thickly sliced
- 2 large green bell peppers, seeded and cut into wedges
- 2 large red bell peppers, seeded and cut into wedges
- 3 large onions, cut into wedges
- ½ cup white wine
- ½ cup chicken stock
- 1 teaspoon Italian seasoning
- salt and freshly ground black pepper to taste

Directions

1. Preheat oven to 400 degrees F (200 degrees C).

2. Heat 2 teaspoons olive oil in a large skillet over medium heat, and cook and stir the sausage until browned, 5 to 10 minutes. Transfer cooked sausage to a large baking dish.

3. Pour 1/4 cup of olive oil into the skillet, and cook potatoes, stirring occasionally, until browned, about 10 minutes. Place the potatoes into the baking dish, leaving some oil in the skillet.

4. Cook and stir green and red peppers and onions in the hot skillet until they are beginning to soften, about 5 minutes. Add the vegetables to the baking dish.

5. Pour wine and chicken stock over the vegetables and sausage, and sprinkle with Italian seasoning, salt, and pepper. Gently stir sausage, potatoes, and vegetables together.

6. Bake in the preheated oven until hot and bubbling, 20 to 25 minutes. Serve hot.

5. Baked Italian Chicken Dinner

Prep Time: 15 mins

Total Time: 1 hr

Servings: 4

Ingredients

- 1 pound skinless, boneless chicken breast, cut into cubes
- 1 (10 ounce) package frozen broccoli
- 4 potatoes, diced
- ¼ cup butter, melted
- 1 (.7 ounce) package Italian dressing mix

Directions

1. Preheat the oven to 350 degrees F (175 degrees C). Spray a 13x9-inch baking dish with cooking spray.
2. Layer chicken, broccoli, and potatoes evenly into the prepared baking dish in the order listed. Drizzle melted butter over the top. Sprinkle with Italian dressing mix.

3. Bake in the preheated oven until chicken is cooked through and potatoes are tender, 45 to 60 minutes.

6. Sweet and Spicy Jerk Shrimp

Prep Time: 20 mins

Total Time: 35 mins

Servings: 4

Ingredients

- 1 ½ pounds large shrimp in shells
- 1 (20 ounce) can pineapple slices packed in 100% juice, drained, and cut into 2-inch pieces
- 2 red bell peppers, cut into thin strips
- 1 large red onion, sliced
- 1 jalapeno pepper - halved lengthwise, seeded, and sliced
- 2 tablespoons olive oil
- 1 tablespoon Jamaican jerk seasoning
- ½ cup chopped fresh cilantro
- 2 cups hot cooked brown rice
- 1 lime, cut into wedges

Directions

1. Preheat the oven to 425 degrees F (220 degrees C). Line two 10x15-inch baking pans with foil.

2. Peel and devein shrimp, leaving tails intact if desired. Rinse shrimp and pat dry.

3. Gently toss shrimp together with pineapple, bell peppers, red onion, jalapeno, oil, and jerk seasoning in a large bowl. Divide mixture between the prepared pans.

4. Roast in the preheated oven until shrimp are opaque, about 15 minutes.

5. Sprinkle with cilantro and serve with brown rice and lime wedges.

7. Greek Flank Steak and Veggie Salad

Prep Time: 25 mins

Total Time: 2 hrs 56 mins

Servings: 6

Ingredients

- 2 pounds flank steak
- 6 tablespoons extra-virgin olive oil
- ¼ cup fresh lemon juice
- 2 tablespoons Worcestershire sauce
- 4 cloves garlic, minced
- 2 teaspoons ground oregano
- 1 teaspoon kosher salt
- ¼ teaspoon black pepper
- 1 (15 ounce) can chickpeas, drained and rinsed
- 1 ½ cups cherry tomatoes, halved
- 1 English cucumber, chopped
- 1 red onion, chopped
- 8 cups chopped romaine lettuce
- 1 cup crumbled feta cheese
- ¼ cup chopped fresh parsley

Directions

1. Put steak in a large resealable plastic bag. Whisk olive oil, lemon juice, Worcestershire sauce, garlic, oregano, salt, and pepper in a small bowl. Reserve 1/2 cup marinade for vegetables; pour remainder over steak and turn to coat. Seal bag. Chill at least 2 hours or up to 12 hours.

2. Preheat oven to 450 degrees F (230 degrees C). Place 1 rack in center position and another 4 inches from broiler. Line a baking sheet with aluminum foil and spray with cooking spray.

3. Toss chickpeas, tomatoes, cucumber, and onion with reserved 1/2 cup marinade on the prepared baking sheet and spread in an even layer.

4. Roast on center rack until vegetables begin to pucker and brown, 15 to 20 minutes.

5. Remove baking sheet from oven and turn oven to broil. Push vegetables to the middle of the pan. Remove steak from marinade, allowing excess liquid to drip off, brush off garlic, and set on top of vegetables. Discard marinade.

6. Broil steak on top rack, flipping once, until it begins to char and an instant-read thermometer inserted into thickest part registers 125 degrees F for rare or 135 degrees F for medium-rare, 3 to 5 minutes per side.

7. Cover loosely with foil and let rest 10 minutes before slicing steak thinly across the grain. Serve warm steak and vegetables with pan juices over romaine, sprinkled with feta cheese and parsley.

Prep Time: 35 mins

Total Time: 1 hr 20 mins

Servings: 8

Ingredients

- ⅓ cup vegetable oil
- 2 teaspoons chili powder
- 1 teaspoon dried oregano
- ½ teaspoon garlic powder
- ½ teaspoon onion powder
- ½ teaspoon ground cumin
- ½ teaspoon salt
- ¼ teaspoon ground black pepper
- 1 pinch ground cayenne pepper
- 1 ½ pounds chicken tenders, quartered
- 4 cups sliced bell peppers, any color
- 1 onion, sliced
- ¼ cup chopped fresh cilantro
- ½ lime, juiced

Directions

1. Combine vegetable oil, chili powder, oregano, garlic, onion, cumin, salt, pepper, and cayenne pepper in a large resealable plastic bag. Add chicken tenders, bell peppers, and onion; shake to mix.

2. Marinate chicken mixture in the refrigerator, 30 minutes to 2 hours.

3. Preheat oven to 400 degrees F (200 degrees C). Line a rimmed sheet pan with aluminum foil.

4. Spread chicken mixture onto prepared pan.

5. Roast in the preheated oven, stirring halfway through, until chicken is no longer pink and bell peppers soften, 15 to 20 minutes.

6. Sprinkle cilantro and pour lime juice over chicken mixture; toss to distribute.

Prep Time: 15 mins

Total Time: 40 mins

Servings: 4

Ingredients

- ½ cup panko bread crumbs
- ¼ cup freshly grated Parmesan cheese
- 4 (5 ounce) bone-in, skin on chicken thighs
- ¼ cup melted butter
- 2 tablespoons Dijon mustard
- 1 ½ pounds tri-color baby potatoes (red, gold, and purple)
- 1 pound fresh green beans, trimmed
- 1 teaspoon dried thyme
- freshly cracked salt and pepper to taste

Directions

1. Preheat the oven to 425 degrees F (220 degrees C). Line a large sheet pan or jelly roll pan with

aluminum foil and coat with nonstick cooking spray.

2. Mix bread crumbs and Parmesan cheese in a small bowl. Set aside.

3. Place chicken thighs on the prepared baking sheet. Stir together butter and Dijon in a large bowl. Brush the tops of the chicken thighs with some of the butter-Dijon mixture.

4. Add potatoes and green beans to the bowl and toss in the remaining butter-Dijon mixture. Spread vegetables around the chicken onto the baking sheet in an even layer. Season everything with thyme, salt, and pepper. Press the bread crumb mixture onto the top of the chicken thighs.

5. Bake in the preheated oven until chicken is no longer pink at the bone and the juices run clear and the potatoes can be pierced easily with a fork, 25 to 30 minutes. An instant-read thermometer inserted near the bone should read 165 degrees F (74 degrees C).

10. Earth, Sea and Fire Salmon

Prep Time: 15 mins

Total Time: 1 hr

Servings: 8

Ingredients

- 2 tablespoons olive oil
- 4 (8 ounce) salmon fillets
- 4 medium potatoes, peeled and sliced
- 2 large red onions, sliced into rings
- 1 jarred roasted red pepper, drained and cut into strips
- 8 ounces portobello mushrooms
- 1 tablespoon fresh lemon juice
- salt and pepper to taste
- 1 teaspoon sesame oil

Directions

1. Preheat the oven to 350 degrees. Coat the bottom of a 9x13 inch baking dish generously with olive oil.

2. Arrange potato slices in a layer on the bottom of the baking dish. Season with a little salt and pepper. Place a layer of onions over the potatoes, then a layer of roasted peppers, seasoning each layer with salt and pepper as desired. Place salmon fillets over the vegetables in the dish, and season with lemon juice, salt and pepper. Place whole mushrooms over the fillets, and drizzle them with sesame oil.

3. Bake for 45 minutes in the preheated oven. Fish should flake easily with a fork, and potatoes should be tender.

11. Chicken, Sausage, Peppers, and Potatoes

Prep Time: 20 mins

Total Time: 1 hr 30 mins

Servings: 6

Ingredients

- 4 large links hot Italian sausage
- 2 tablespoons olive oil, divided
- 6 bone-in, skin on chicken thighs
- ½ pound assorted sweet peppers, seeded
- 1 small red onion, sliced
- ½ yellow onion, sliced
- 4 large Yukon Gold potatoes, quartered
- 2 teaspoons dried Italian herbs
- 2 teaspoons kosher salt, plus more as needed
- Freshly ground black pepper to taste
- 1 tablespoon Chopped fresh Italian parsley

Directions

1. Preheat oven to 450 degrees F (230 degrees C).

2. Heat olive oil in a skillet over medium heat. Cook sausage links until browned and oil begins to render, about 3 minutes per side. While sausages are cooking, pierce them lightly here and there with the tip of a sharp knife so some fats and juices are released. Remove from heat and let cool slightly.

3. When sausages are cool enough to handle, cut them into serving pieces, about 2-inch slices. Transfer back to pan along with any accumulated juices from the cutting board.

4. Cut two slashes down to the bone on the skin side of each chicken thigh.

5. Depending on the size of the peppers, halve or quarter them and place in a large mixing bowl. Add the sliced red and yellow onions and potato chunks. Add chicken thighs and sausage pieces with pan juices.

6. Season with kosher salt, black pepper, and Italian herbs. Drizzle with a tablespoon of olive oil.

7. Mix with your hands until all ingredients are coated in oil, 3 or 4 minutes. Transfer to large, heavy-duty roasting pan. Evenly space the

chicken thighs skin side up. Position potatoes near the top.

8. Place in preheated oven until chicken is cooked through and everything is caramelized, about 1 hour. An instant-read thermometer inserted near the bone should read 165 degrees F (74 degrees C). Sprinkle with chopped fresh Italian parsley, if desired.

Prep Time: 20 mins

Total Time: 50 mins

Servings: 4

Ingredients

- 1 large head broccoli, cut into florets
- 10 ounces baby potatoes, halved
- 1 large carrot, sliced
- ½ red onion, roughly chopped
- 3 tablespoons olive oil
- 2 tablespoons whole grain mustard
- 2 tablespoons grated Pecorino Romano cheese
- 1 teaspoon dried thyme
- ½ teaspoon dried oregano
- salt and ground black pepper to taste
- 4 mild Italian sausage links

Directions

1. Preheat the oven to 400 degrees F (200 degrees C).

2. Place broccoli, baby potatoes, carrot, and onion in a large bowl. Pour in olive oil, mustard, Pecorino Romano cheese, thyme, oregano, salt, and pepper. Toss well to coat, then spread vegetables in an even layer on a sheet pan. Arrange sausages in the pan, pushing aside the vegetables so that the sausages touch the bottom of the pan.

3. Bake in the preheated oven, flipping sausages and vegetables halfway through until sausages are no longer pink in the center, 30 to 35 minutes. An instant-read thermometer inserted into the center should read 160 degrees F (70 degrees C).

13. Maple-Roasted Chicken Thighs

Prep Time: 20 mins

Total Time: 50 mins

Servings: 4

Ingredients

- 2 tablespoons olive oil, divided
- 2 tablespoons maple syrup
- 1 tablespoon snipped fresh thyme
- ¾ teaspoon salt, divided
- ¾ teaspoon ground black pepper, divided
- 1 pound sweet potatoes, peeled and cut into 1-inch wedges
- 1 pound Brussels sprouts, trimmed and halved
- 4 bone-in chicken thighs
- ¼ cup chopped toasted pecans
- ¼ cup chopped dried cranberries

Directions

1. Preheat the oven to 425 degrees F (220 degrees C). Line a 10x15-inch baking pan with foil.

2. Whisk 1 teaspoon olive oil, maple syrup, thyme, 1/4 teaspoon salt, and 1/4 teaspoon pepper together in a small bowl. Set aside.

3. Toss sweet potatoes and Brussels sprouts together in a large bowl with 2 teaspoons olive oil, 1/4 teaspoon salt, and 1/4 teaspoon pepper.

4. Brush chicken with remaining olive oil and sprinkle with remaining salt and pepper. Arrange chicken, smooth sides down, in the center of the prepared pan. Arrange vegetables around chicken.

5. Roast in the preheated oven for 15 minutes.

6. Turn chicken over; brush it, sweet potatoes, and Brussels sprouts with maple syrup mixture. Continue to roast until potatoes are tender and an instant-read thermometer inserted into thickest parts of the chicken registers 175 degrees F (80 degrees C), about 15 minutes. Sprinkle with pecans and cranberries.

14. Easy Vegan Sheet Pan Roasted Cauliflower, Tomatoes, and Garbanzo Beans

Prep Time: 10 mins

Total Time: 35 mins

Servings: 2

Ingredients

- 1 tablespoon olive oil
- 2 cloves garlic, minced
- ½ teaspoon salt
- ¼ teaspoon ground black pepper
- 4 cups sliced cauliflower
- 2 cups cherry tomatoes
- 1 (15 ounce) can garbanzo beans, drained
- 1 lime, cut into wedges
- 1 tablespoon chopped fresh cilantro

Directions

1. Preheat oven to 450 degrees F (230 degrees C). Line a baking sheet with aluminum foil and grease with cooking spray.

2. Combine olive oil, garlic, salt, and pepper in a bowl. Add cauliflower, tomatoes, and garbanzo beans; toss until well coated. Spread in a single layer on the prepared baking sheet. Add lime wedges.

3. Roast in the preheated oven until vegetables are caramelized, about 25 minutes. Remove lime wedges and top with fresh cilantro.

15. Sheet Pan Beef Fajitas

Prep Time: 20 mins

Total Time: 40 mins

Servings: 6

Ingredients

- 2 medium bell peppers, sliced
- 1 medium onion, sliced
- 1 tablespoon olive oil, divided
- 1 ½ teaspoons salt, divided
- 1 teaspoon chili powder, divided
- ¾ teaspoon garlic powder
- ¾ teaspoon ground black pepper, divided
- ½ teaspoon ground cumin, divided
- 1 (1 1/2-pound) flank steak
- 2 medium limes, quartered
- 6 (6 inch) flour tortillas, warmed

Directions

1. Preheat the oven to 450 degrees F (230 degrees C). Line a sheet pan with foil.

2. Combine bell peppers, onion, 2 teaspoons oil, 3/4 teaspoon salt, 1/2 teaspoon chili powder, garlic powder, 1/4 teaspoon pepper, and 1/4 teaspoon cumin on the prepared pan; toss to coat. Spread veggie mixture around the sides of the pan creating a space in the center.

3. Place flank steak in center of pan and brush with remaining 1 teaspoon oil. Sprinkle steak with remaining salt, chili powder, pepper, and cumin and rub to evenly coat.

4. Bake in the preheated oven until veggies are tender and browned around the edges and steak is beginning to firm and is hot and slightly pink in the center, 12 to 14 minutes, or to desired degree of doneness. An instant-read thermometer inserted into the center of the steak should read 140 degrees F (60 degrees C) for medium.

5. Transfer steak to a cutting board and rest, 5 to 10 minutes.

6. Thinly slice steak and return to the sheet pan. Add lime wedges and serve with tortillas.

16. Sheet Pan Salmon and Bell Pepper Dinner

Prep Time: 20 mins

Total Time: 30 mins

Servings: 4

Ingredients

- 2 tablespoons olive oil
- 4 (3 ounce) fillets salmon fillets
- 2 red bell peppers, chopped
- 1 yellow bell pepper, chopped
- 1 onion, sliced
- Sauce:
- 6 tablespoons lemon juice
- 3 tablespoons olive oil
- 2 tablespoons water
- 1 tablespoon maple syrup
- 5 cloves garlic
- 1 ½ teaspoons salt
- 1 ½ teaspoons red pepper flakes
- 1 teaspoon ground cumin
- ½ bunch fresh parsley, chopped

- 1 lemon, sliced

Directions

1. Preheat oven to 400 degrees F (200 degrees C). Grease a sheet pan with 2 tablespoons olive oil.
2. Place salmon fillets, red and yellow bell peppers, and onion on the prepared sheet pan.
3. Combine lemon juice, 3 tablespoons olive oil, water, maple syrup, garlic, salt, red pepper flakes, cumin, and parsley in a small bowl. Drizzle 2/3 of the sauce over the ingredients on the sheet pan.
4. Bake in the preheated oven until salmon is cooked through and flakes easily with a fork, 10 to 15 minutes.
5. Serve with lemon slices and remaining sauce.

17. Italian Chicken Sausage and Peppers

Prep Time: 25 mins

Total Time: 1 hr 5 mins

Servings: 4

Ingredients

- 1 red bell pepper, cut into 1-inch pieces
- 1 yellow bell pepper, cut into 1-inch pieces
- 1 orange bell pepper, cut into 1-inch pieces
- 1 green bell pepper, cut into 1-inch pieces
- 1 large sweet onion, cut into thin wedges
- 2 cups grape tomatoes
- 2 tablespoons olive oil, divided
- 1 tablespoon balsamic vinegar
- ¼ teaspoon Italian seasoning
- ¼ teaspoon salt, divided
- ¼ teaspoon ground black pepper, divided
- 1 (8 ounce) baguette, thinly sliced
- 1 (12 ounce) package cooked Italian chicken sausage, sliced diagonally into thirds
- 1 tablespoon snipped fresh oregano

Directions

1. Arrange 2 racks in middle and upper thirds of oven and preheat to 425 degrees F (220 degrees C). Line two 10x15-inch baking pans with foil.

2. Toss bell peppers, onion, and tomatoes together in a large bowl with 1 tablespoon oil, balsamic vinegar, Italian seasoning, 1/8 teaspoon salt, and 1/8 teaspoon black pepper. Transfer to one of the prepared pans.

3. Roast in the preheated oven for 30 minutes.

4. Meanwhile, drizzle bread slices with remaining olive oil and sprinkle with remaining salt and black pepper. Arrange on the other prepared pan.

5. Remove the vegetables from the oven; push to one side of the pan. Add sausage to the exposed portion of the pan.

6. Roast until vegetables are tender and sausage is heated through, 10 to 15 minutes more, adding the pan with bread in the last 5 minutes of roasting time. Sprinkle vegetables and sausage with oregano and serve with bread.

18. Baked Chicken Breasts and Vegetables

Prep Time: 20 mins

Total Time: 50 mins

Servings: 4

Ingredients

- 4 skinless, boneless chicken breast halves
- 8 carrots, sliced into 1/2-inch rounds
- 8 stalks celery, chopped
- 8 green onions, chopped
- 4 green bell peppers, sliced
- ¼ cup chopped fresh flat-leaf parsley
- ½ cup olive oil
- 1 teaspoon Italian seasoning
- 1 teaspoon chili powder
- 1 teaspoon lemon pepper
- 1 teaspoon salt
- 4 pinches freshly ground black pepper, or to taste

Directions

1. Preheat the oven to 375 degrees F (190 degrees C).

2. Arrange chicken breasts on a baking sheet; spread carrots, celery, green onion, bell pepper, and parsley around chicken. Drizzle olive oil over chicken and vegetables; season with Italian seasoning, chili powder, lemon pepper, salt, and black pepper.

3. Bake in the preheated oven until chicken is no longer pink in the center and juices run clear, about 30 minutes. An instant-read thermometer inserted into the center should read at least 165 degrees F (74 degrees C).

19. Apple Slab Pie

Prep Time: 30 mins

Total Time: 1 hr 30 mins

Servings: 15

Ingredients

- 1 ½ cups all-purpose flour
- 1 ½ tablespoons white sugar
- ½ cup shortening
- ¼ teaspoon salt
- ½ teaspoon baking powder
- 2 egg yolks, beaten
- 4 tablespoons water
- 8 apples - peeled, cored and cut into thin wedges
- 2 tablespoons lemon juice
- 2 tablespoons all-purpose flour
- 1 ¾ cups white sugar
- ½ teaspoon ground cinnamon
- 2 tablespoons butter
- 1 cup all-purpose flour
- 1 teaspoon ground cinnamon

- ⅔ cup brown sugar

- ⅔ cup butter

Directions

1. Preheat oven to 350 degrees F (175 degrees C.) In a large bowl, combine flour sugar, salt and baking powder. Cut in shortening until mixture resembles coarse crumbs. Mix egg yolk and water together and mix into flour until it forms a ball. Roll out to fit the bottom of a 10x15 inch pan.

2. In a large bowl, combine apples, lemon juice, 2 tablespoons flour, sugar and cinnamon. Pour filling into pie crust and dot with 2 tablespoons butter.

3. In a medium bowl, combine 1 cup flour, 1 teaspoon cinnamon, 2/3 cup brown sugar and 2/3 cup butter. Cut in the butter until crumbly, then sprinkle over apples.

4. Bake in the preheated oven for 60 minutes, or until topping is golden brown.

20. Apple Pot Pies

Prep Time: 10 mins

Total Time: 30 mins

Servings: 12

Ingredients

- 1 ⅓ cups brown sugar
- 2 tablespoons ground cinnamon
- 1 tablespoon butter
- 2 teaspoons honey
- 8 small Golden Delicious apples, peeled and cut into small pieces
- 1 refrigerated pie crust

Directions

1. Preheat the oven to 375 degrees F (190 degrees C).
2. Combine sugar, cinnamon, butter, and honey in a medium saucepan over medium heat; stir. Mix in apples. Cook until softened, about 10 minutes.

3. Meanwhile, cut pie crust into 12 rounds to fit the cups of a cupcake pan and press into cups to make crusts.

4. Fill crusts 3/4 full with cooked apple mixture.

5. Bake in the preheated oven until crust edges are golden brown and not doughy, 10 to 15 minutes. Let cool before serving.

21. Apple Upside-Down Cake

Prep Time: 20 mins

Total Time: 1 hr 25 mins

Servings: 12

Ingredients

- 1 ½ cups brown sugar, or more to taste
- 3 tablespoons ground cinnamon, divided
- 5 medium apples - peeled, cored, and sliced
- 4 cups all-purpose flour
- 1 ½ cups unsweetened apple juice
- 1 ½ cups white sugar
- 1 cup butter, softened
- 4 eggs
- ½ cup milk
- 1 tablespoon vanilla extract
- 2 teaspoons baking powder
- 2 teaspoons salt

Directions

1. Preheat the oven to 350 degrees F (175 degrees C).

2. Cover the bottom of a 10x15-inch baking pan with brown sugar and 2 tablespoons cinnamon. Layer apple slices on top.

3. Place flour, apple juice, white sugar, butter, eggs, milk, remaining 1 tablespoon cinnamon, vanilla extract, baking powder, and salt in the bowl of a stand mixer fitted with the paddle attachment. Mix until completely smooth, 5 to 10 minutes; the longer you mix, the fluffier the cake will be.

4. Pour batter over apples in the baking pan, making sure they are evenly covered.

5. Bake in the preheated oven until a toothpick inserted into the center comes out clean, 45 to 55 minutes. Cool for 20 to 30 minutes. Place a large serving dish over the cake and carefully flip over.

Prep Time: 30 mins

Total Time: 1 hr 18 mins

Servings: 60

Ingredients

- 2 cups all-purpose flour
- 1 teaspoon baking soda
- 1 teaspoon ground cinnamon
- 1 teaspoon ground cloves
- ½ teaspoon ground nutmeg
- ½ teaspoon salt
- ½ cup softened butter
- 1 ½ cups packed brown sugar
- 1 egg, beaten
- 1 cup chopped walnuts
- 1 cup chopped apples
- 1 cup raisins
- ⅔ cup confectioners' sugar
- 1 tablespoon milk

Directions

1. Preheat oven to 350 degrees F (175 degrees C). Line cookie sheets with parchment paper.

2. In a medium bowl, sift together flour, baking soda, cinnamon, cloves, nutmeg, and salt. In a large mixing bowl, cream butter until light and fluffy. Mix in sugar and egg. Stir in flour mixture, and mix thoroughly. Fold in nuts, apples, and raisins.

3. Drop by rounded teaspoon onto prepared cookie sheets about 1 1/2 inches apart. Bake for 12 to 14 minutes. Cool on wire rack.

4. In a small bowl, mix confectioners' sugar with milk to make a thin glaze. Drizzle over cooled cookies.

Prep Time: 20 mins

Total Time: 1 hr 5 mins

Servings: 6

Ingredients

- 6 medium baking apples, peeled and cored
- 2 cups all-purpose flour
- 2 ½ teaspoons baking powder
- ½ teaspoon salt
- ⅔ cup shortening
- ½ cup milk
- 3 cups brown sugar, divided
- 1 teaspoon ground cinnamon
- 2 cups water
- ¼ cup butter
- ¼ teaspoon ground nutmeg

Directions

1. Preheat the oven to 375 degrees F (190 degrees C). Spray a 9x13-inch baking dish with cooking spray.

2. Set apples aside in a cold water bath while you prepare the dough.

3. Combine flour, baking powder, and salt in a medium mixing bowl. Add shortening and cut together with a pastry blender or a fork until crumbly. Add milk and stir until dough comes together.

4. Combine 1 cup brown sugar and cinnamon in another bowl. Separate dough into six equal portions and roll out to about 1/4-inch thickness. Place an apple in the center of each dough portion and fill the core with the cinnamon-sugar mixture. Wrap each apple in dough and place into the prepared pan.

5. Combine remaining brown sugar, water, butter, and nutmeg in a medium saucepan over medium-high heat. Cook until sugar is dissolved and butter

is melted, about 5 minutes. Pour syrup over dumplings.

6. Bake in the preheated oven until dough is golden brown and apples are soft, about 40 minutes.

24. Apple Frangipane Cake

Prep Time: 15 mins

Total Time: 2 hrs 15 mins

Servings: 12

Ingredients

- ½ cup unsalted butter, softened
- 6 tablespoons unsalted butter, softened
- 1 (7 ounce) package almond paste
- 1 cup white sugar
- 1 teaspoon vanilla bean paste
- 5 large eggs
- 1 cup sifted cake flour
- ½ teaspoon kosher salt
- 2 medium Apples, raw
- 1 tablespoon unsalted butter, melted
- 1 tablespoon white sugar
- ¼ cup powdered sugar, or to taste
- 2 tablespoons toasted sliced almonds, or to taste

Directions

1. Preheat the oven to 350 degrees F (175 degrees
    C). Grease and flour a 9-inch round springform
    pan.

2. Beat 1/2 cup plus 6 tablespoons softened butter,
    almond paste, and 1 cup sugar at low speed with a
    stand mixer fitted with the paddle attachment,
    until combined. Increase speed to medium-high
    and beat until smooth, light, and fluffy, 3 to 4
    minutes. Beat in vanilla bean paste; add eggs, 1 at
    a time, and beat until completely combined after
    each addition. Gently fold in flour and salt with a
    rubber spatula until just combined.

3. Spoon mixture into the prepared springform pan.
    Arrange apples slices over top of batter; brush
    apples with melted butter and sprinkle with 1
    tablespoon sugar.

4. Bake in the preheated oven until browned and a
    wooden pick inserted in the center comes out
    clean, 50 to 55 minutes. Remove to a wire rack
    and cool for 10 minutes. Remove sides of pan and
    cool completely, about 1 hour. Dust top of cake

with powdered sugar and sprinkle with toasted
sliced almonds.

25. Torta di Mele Italian Apple Cake

Prep Time: 20 mins

Total Time: 50 mins

Servings: 8

Ingredients

- 2 tablespoons unseasoned bread crumbs, or as needed
- ½ cup unsalted butter, melted
- ½ cup white sugar
- 1 vanilla bean, split and scraped
- 2 eggs
- 1 ⅛ cups all-purpose flour
- 1 teaspoon baking powder
- 1 pinch salt
- 1 tablespoon milk, or as needed
- 2 pounds Granny Smith apples, peeled, cored and sliced thin
- ¼ cup unsalted butter, cubed
- ¼ cup white sugar

Directions

1. Preheat the oven to 375 degrees F (190 degrees C). Grease a pie plate and dust with bread crumbs

2. Combine melted butter, 1/2 cup sugar, and vanilla bean seeds in a bowl. Add eggs and stir to combine. Mix flour, baking powder, and salt in a bowl and add to butter mixture. Add milk if batter is too thick

3. Pour batter into the prepared pie plate. Distribute apple slices in a thick layer on top of the batter. Dot with cubed butter and sprinkle with 1/4 cup sugar.

4. Bake in the preheated oven until a toothpick inserted into the center comes out clean, 30 to 45 minutes. Cool on a wire rack for 5 minutes. Run a table knife around the edges to loosen. Invert carefully onto a serving plate or cooling rack. Let cool completely.

26. Apple Crisp Cheesecake

Prep Time: 20 mins

Total Time: 5 hrs

Servings: 8

Ingredients

- 1 teaspoon lemon juice, or as needed
- 1 cup water, or as desired
- 2 medium Granny Smith apples - peeled, cored, and sliced, or more to taste
- ⅓ cup white sugar
- ½ teaspoon ground cinnamon
- 1 (8 ounce) package cream cheese, softened
- ¼ cup white sugar
- 1 large egg
- ½ teaspoon vanilla extract
- 1 (10 inch) graham cracker crust
- ⅓ cup quick-cooking oats

Directions

1. Preheat oven to 375 degrees F (190 degrees C).

2. Stir lemon juice and water together in a bowl; add apples to stop browning process. Whisk 1/3 cup sugar and cinnamon together in a separate bowl.

3. Beat cream cheese and 1/4 cup sugar together in a bowl using an electric mixer until smooth; add egg and vanilla extract and mix until evenly combined.

4. Drain apples and transfer to the graham cracker crust. Sprinkle cinnamon-sugar mixture and oats over apples. Pour cream cheese mixture over apple mixture.

5. Bake in the preheated oven until top is just beginning to brown, about 40 minutes. Cool on a wire rack, 1 to 2 hours. Refrigerate until completely set, 3 to 4 hours.

27. Sheet Pan Sausage and Seasonal Vegetables

Prep Time: 10 mins

Total Time: 30 mins

Servings: 4

Ingredients

- 1 pound peeled and cubed butternut squash
- 1 pound pork sausage, sliced
- ½ pound peeled and sliced carrots
- 3 cups shredded red cabbage
- 1 cup sliced onion
- 3 tablespoons minced garlic
- 2 tablespoons vegetable oil
- 1 tablespoon salt
- 2 teaspoons ground black pepper
- 1 teaspoon herbes de Provence

Directions

1. Preheat the oven to 400 degrees F (200 degrees C). Line a roasting pan or large baking dish with aluminum foil.

2. Add squash, sausage, carrots, cabbage, and onion to the prepared pan. Toss with garlic, oil, salt, pepper, and herbes de Provence.

3. Roast in the preheated oven until vegetables are tender and sausage is browned, about 20 minutes.

28. Apple-Cinnamon Burrito

Prep Time: 5 mins

Total Time: 25 mins

Servings: 1

Ingredients

- 1 medium apple - peeled, cored, and sliced
- 2 teaspoons water
- ½ tablespoon unsalted butter
- 2 teaspoons brown sugar
- ½ teaspoon ground cinnamon
- 1 (8 inch) flour tortilla
- 2 scoops vanilla ice cream

Directions

1. Place apple slices and water in a microwave-safe bowl and cover tightly with plastic wrap. Microwave on high power until apple slices are soft, about 3 minutes.

2. Mix butter, brown sugar, and cinnamon in another microwave-safe bowl. Microwave in 30-

second intervals, stirring after each interval, until melted and the consistency is of a thick liquid. Spread on tortilla and lay apple down the middle. Place in the refrigerator until cool, about 15 minutes.

3. Remove from the refrigerator and place ice cream on top of apples. Wrap tortilla as you would wrap a burrito.

Servings: 12

Ingredients

- 1 ½ cups vegetable oil
- 3 eggs
- 1 cup packed brown sugar
- 2 teaspoons vanilla extract
- 1 teaspoon baking soda
- 1 teaspoon salt
- 3 cups all-purpose flour
- 1 cup chopped walnuts
- 4 cups chopped apples
- 1 cup packed brown sugar
- ½ cup butter
- ¼ cup heavy whipping cream

Directions

1. Preheat oven to 350 degrees F (175 degrees C). Grease and flour a 9x13 inch pan, or a 10 inch tube pan. Stir the flour, baking soda and salt together and set aside.

2. In a large bowl, cream the oil, eggs, 1 cup brown sugar and 2 teaspoons vanilla. Add the flour mixture and mix well. Stir in the chopped apples and nuts.

3. Pour batter into prepared pan. Bake at 350 degrees F (175 degrees C) for 30 minutes, or until a toothpick inserted into the center of the cake comes out clean.

4. For the Topping: In a saucepan, combine 1 cup brown sugar, 1/2 cup butter and 1/4 cup cream. Bring to a boil, and continue boiling for 3 minutes. Cool slightly and pour over warm cake.

30. Warm Apple Buttermilk Custard Pie

Servings: 8

Ingredients

- 1 (9 inch) pie shell
- ¼ cup butter
- 2 tart apples - peeled, cored and sliced
- ½ cup white sugar
- ½ teaspoon ground cinnamon
- ¼ cup butter, softened
- 1 ⅓ cups white sugar
- 4 eggs
- 1 teaspoon vanilla extract
- 2 tablespoons all-purpose flour
- ¾ cup buttermilk
- ¼ cup white sugar
- ¼ cup packed brown sugar
- ½ cup all-purpose flour
- ¼ teaspoon ground cinnamon
- 3 tablespoons butter

Directions

1. Preheat oven to 300 degrees F (150 degrees C).

2. To Make Apple Filling: Melt 1/4 cup butter or margarine in skillet over medium heat. Add apple, 1/2 cup white sugar, and 1/2 teaspoon cinnamon. Cook 3 to 5 minutes, until tender. Set aside.

3. To Make Buttermilk Custard: In a large mixing bowl combine 1/4 cup softened butter or margarine with 1 1/3 cups white sugar. Beat until creamy. Add eggs one at a time, beating until yellow disappears. Mix in vanilla, then 2 tablespoons flour. Combine thoroughly, then pour in buttermilk, beating until smooth.

4. Fit pastry into pie pan and prick with a fork. Spoon apple mixture into crust, then pour buttermilk custard over it.

5. Place in preheated oven and bake for 30 minutes.

6. To Make Streusel Topping: While pie is baking, combine 1/4 cup white sugar, brown sugar, 1/2 cup flour, and 1/4 teaspoon cinnamon in a small bowl. Cut in 3 tablespoons butter or margarine until mixture is crumbly.

7. Remove pie from oven after 30 minutes and sprinkle streusel topping over custard. Return to oven and bake for an additional 40 to 50 minutes, until a knife inserted in center comes out clean. Let stand 1 hour before serving.